PREGNACY REVELATIONS

Unraveling the Web of Intriguing Facts Surrounding Expectant Mothers

ELLIOT BALDWIN

Foreword

Welcome to a journey that delves deep into the captivating and wondrous world of expectant mothers. In "Pregnancy Revelations," we embark on an expedition to unravel the intricate tapestry of facts, emotions, and experiences that surround the miracle of life. This book is a celebration of the resplendent journey that women embark upon when they embrace the gift of pregnancy. Within these pages, we will explore the scientific marvels that underpin pregnancy, tracing the remarkable transformation of a tiny seed into a beautiful being, nurturing the potential for boundless wonders.

Drawing upon the latest research, time-honored wisdom, and heartwarming anecdotes, "Pregnancy Revelations" will act as your trusted companion. Whether you are an expectant mother, a partner, a family member, or a friend, this book seeks to empower and enlighten, providing insights into the unique challenges and joys that accompany this miraculous phase of life.

Through each chapter, you will explore the profound connections forged between the mother and her unborn child. You will find practical guidance, fostering a nurturing environment for the little one, and fostering maternal well-being.

This book does not shy away from the challenges expectant mothers may face, acknowledging that while pregnancy is a miraculous gift, it can also be accompanied by uncertainties and complexities. Yet, it serves as a beacon of strength, providing insights to navigate the stormy seas, assuring you that you are not alone in this voyage. It is my hope that "Pregnancy Revelations" will not only equip you with knowledge but also inspire a deeper appreciation for the unparalleled strength and resilience of mothers-to-be.

I extend my heartfelt gratitude to every individual who contributed to this exploration of motherhood, as well as to each reader who seeks to understand, support, and cherish the profound experience of pregnancy.

Elliot Baldwin

Author of "Pregnancy Revelations"

Contents

Copyright © 2023 by Elliot Baldwin 2

Foreword 3

Introduction: Embarking on the Journey of Motherhood 7

Chapter 1: The Wonders of Conception and Early Pregnancy 9

1.1 The Miracle of Fertilization: The Dance of the Egg and Sperm 9

1.2 Nesting Instincts: The Intricate Process of Implantation 11

1.3 Double Delight: Unveiling the Mysteries of Twin Pregnancies 12

1.4 From Zygote to Embryo: The Remarkable Stages of Early Development 13

1.5 The Surprising Role of Hormones: Pregnancy's Chemical Symphony 14

Chapter 2: Mind and Body Transformations 16

2.1 The Pregnancy Glow: Unraveling the Secrets Behind Radiant Skin 16

2.2 From Head to Toe: How Pregnancy Affects Your Body 17

2.3 Cravings and Aversions: The Unpredictable Culinary Adventures 17

2.4 Hormonal Rollercoaster: Understanding Emotional Changes 18

2.5 Memory Lapses and "Baby Brain": The Cognitive Impact of Pregnancy 19

Chapter 3: Nourishing Two Lives: The Importance of Diet During Pregnancy 20

3.1 Building a Strong Foundation: The Essential Nutrients for Expectant Mothers 20

3.2 Eating for Two: Dispelling Myths and Embracing Healthy Habits 21

3.3 Food Safety and Pregnancy: A Guide to Making Safe Choices 22

3.4 Managing Weight Gain: Striking a Balance for Mom and Baby 23

3.5 Dealing with Pregnancy Cravings: Satisfying Urges Without Compromising Health 24

Chapter 4: Fascinating Facts about the Growing Bump 25

4.1 The Marvel of Stretch Marks: Science Behind the Lines 25

4.2 It's Kicking! The Thrilling World of Fetal Movement 26

4.3 The Mystery of Belly Button Popping Out 27

4.4 Pregnancy Dreams and Their Symbolism 28

4.5 Carrying High or Low: Debunking Belly Position Myths 29

Chapter 5: Navigating the Ups and Downs of Pregnancy **30**

5.1 Morning Sickness: Causes, Remedies, and Myths 30

4.2 The Second Trimester: Golden Period of Pregnancy 31

4.3 Heartburn and Indigestion: Taming the Fire Within 32

4.4 Sleeping Woes: Finding Comfort in the Land of Nod 33

4.5 The Joys and Challenges of the Third Trimester 33

Chapter 6: Unveiling Gender and Genetic Surprises **35**

6.1 From Pink to Blue: Exploring the Science of Gender Prediction 35

6.2 Genetic Inheritance: Traits Passed Down to Your Baby 35

6.3 Old Wives' Tales: Fun Predictors of Baby's Gender 36

6.4 Genetic Testing: Insights into Your Baby's Health 37

6.5 Surprise, Surprise! Unveiling Unexpected Genetic Conditions 38

Chapter 7: Preparing for Labor and Beyond **39**

7.1 Braxton Hicks Contractions: False Alarms and Practice Runs 39

7.2 The Art of Breathing: Techniques for Labor and Delivery 40

7.3 Baby's First Cry: Why It's a Magical Sound 42

7.4 The Hormonal Orchestra: The Role of Oxytocin in Labor 43

7.5 Packing Your Hospital Bag: Essentials and Personal Touches 43

Chapter 8: Postpartum Surprises and Joys **46**

8.1 The Fourth Trimester: Adjusting to Life with a Newborn 46

8.2 Baby Blues or Postpartum Depression: Navigating Emotional Changes ... 47

8.3 The Truth About Baby Weight: Losing and Loving Your Postpartum Body ... 48

8.4 Breastfeeding Mysteries: From Supply to Latching 48

8.5 Sleepless Nights and Sweet Smiles: The Rewards of Parenthood ... 49

Conclusion **53**

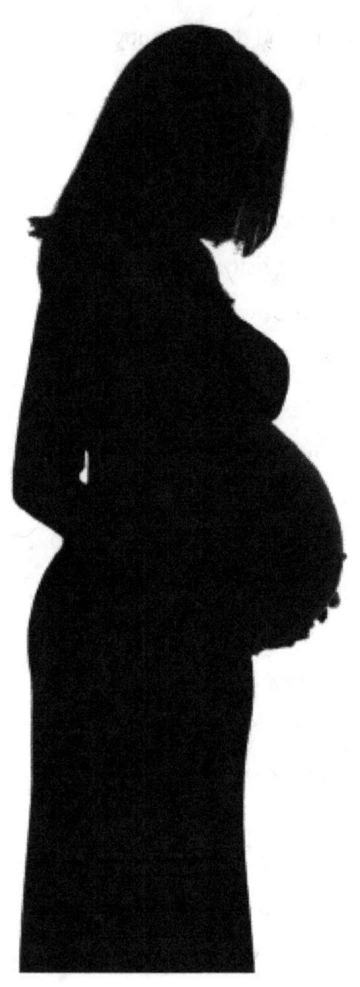

Introduction:

Embarking on the Journey of Motherhood

Becoming a mother is one of the most extraordinary and transformative journeys a woman can embark upon. From the very moment she discovers the tiny seed of life growing within her, a symphony of emotions, questions, and dreams begins to play in her heart. The journey of motherhood is a tapestry woven with threads of wonder, curiosity, and a burning desire to understand the intricate and fascinating facts that surround expectant mothers.

In this age of information, the web of knowledge can often become entangled with myths, half-truths, and conflicting advice, leaving expectant mothers bewildered and overwhelmed. The quest for reliable, evidence-based information is akin to navigating a maze, and it's essential to have a guiding light to help unravel the complexities.

In "Unraveling the Web of Intriguing Facts Surrounding Expectant Mothers," we take you on an enlightening and empowering expedition through the realm of pregnancy and motherhood. Together, we will delve into the science, biology, and psychology behind the miracle of life, as well as explore the cultural, historical, and societal significance of motherhood across the ages.

In this educational and engaging book, we will shine a light on the latest research and discoveries surrounding prenatal care, fetal development, and the well-being of both mother and child. You will discover how a mother's choices and environment can shape the future of her offspring, leaving an indelible mark on generations to come.

But this journey is not solely about scientific facts; it is a celebration of the emotional and spiritual aspects of being an expectant mother. We will explore the profound bond that forms between a mother and her unborn child and the enduring impact it can have on their relationship throughout life.

Moreover, we will address the challenges and triumphs that expectant mothers encounter, navigating the physical and emotional rollercoaster of pregnancy, labor, and postpartum. We aim to provide a comprehensive and compassionate guide to support mothers as they face the joys and uncertainties that accompany this remarkable period in their lives.

As we traverse the chapters of this book, we will debunk myths, challenge stereotypes, and embrace the diversity of experiences that mothers from all walks of life share. We celebrate the strength and resilience of women throughout history who have not only borne children but also shaped societies and cultures.

With each page turned, we will unravel the enigmatic web of pregnancy cravings, superstitions, and rituals, examining how they are interwoven with the rich tapestry of human customs and beliefs. From ancient traditions to modern-day practices, you will be captivated by the kaleidoscope of stories that have shaped the art of motherhood.

So, dear reader, whether you are an expectant mother seeking knowledge and guidance or an enthusiast eager to delve into the wonders of pregnancy, this book is crafted just for you. Join us on this captivating expedition, as we embark on the journey of motherhood together, weaving together the threads of science, history, and emotion to create a tapestry of understanding and empowerment. Let us unravel the web of intriguing facts surrounding expectant mothers, for in doing so, we may discover the true essence of the miracle of life itself.

Chapter 1:

The Wonders of Conception and Early Pregnancy

1.1 The Miracle of Fertilization: The Dance of the Egg and Sperm

At the dawn of human life, a symphony of events takes place inside a woman's body. Each month, as part of her menstrual cycle, an egg prepares itself for the possibility of conception. This egg, no larger than a grain of sand, emerges from one of the ovaries and begins its journey through the intricate labyrinth of the female reproductive system.

Simultaneously, in the depths of the male body, millions of tiny warriors are being created. These are the sperm, each carrying the genetic material that will determine the unique traits of the potential offspring. Their production occurs continuously, ensuring a steady supply of contenders for the momentous race that is yet to come.

When the time is right, nature's clock sets in motion the events that will lead to fertilization. During intercourse, hundreds of millions of sperm are released into the woman's vagina. Their mission is clear - to reach the egg and unite with it, kickstarting the remarkable process of conception.

But this journey is far from easy. The female reproductive tract is a formidable barrier, and the odds are stacked against the sperm. Many will perish in the acidic environment of the vagina, while others may encounter blockages along the way. Yet, these countless casualties are a testament to the importance of this extraordinary quest.

For the lucky few sperm that endure, the race becomes even more intense. The cervix, the gateway between the vagina and the uterus, is a narrow passage that filters out weaker sperm and facilitates the upward movement of the strongest contenders. As they traverse the uterus and enter the fallopian tubes, the sperm's numbers begin to dwindle further.

Meanwhile, the egg waits patiently in one of the fallopian tubes, basking in the anticipation of potential fertilization. Its surface, protected by the zona pellucida, is primed for a fateful encounter. The zona pellucida plays a vital role in selecting the most suitable partner for the egg. Only a sperm with a strong and healthy genetic composition will be able to penetrate this protective layer and continue the journey towards fertilization.

As the remaining sperm reach the egg's vicinity, a final sprint ensues. They release enzymes that aid in breaking down the zona pellucida, ensuring that only one sperm can successfully penetrate and fuse with the egg. The moment of fertilization is nigh.

Finally, one exceptional sperm emerges victorious. As it fuses with the egg, their genetic material combines, culminating in the creation of a single cell that holds the potential to develop into a unique individual. This newly formed cell, called a zygote, represents the very beginning of a human life.

Within hours, the zygote embarks on a series of rapid divisions, transforming into a cluster of cells known as a blastocyst. The blastocyst will continue its journey towards the uterus, where it will seek a suitable spot to implant itself in the uterine lining.

The dance of the egg and sperm sets the stage for the journey of a lifetime – the transformation from a single cell to a fully-formed human being, ready to explore the world. It is a tale of wonder, resilience, and the boundless beauty of life's inception – a testament to the breathtaking miracles that occur within the human body, from the very beginning.

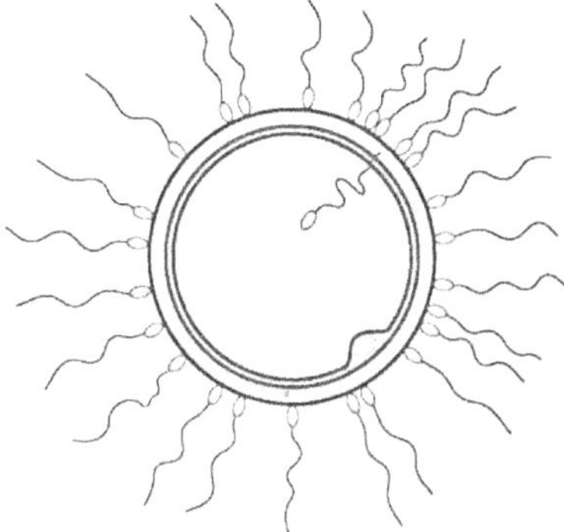

Spermatozoa racing towards the awaiting egg in a quest for fertilization.

1.2   Nesting Instincts: The Intricate Process of Implantation

Once fertilization occurs, a new chapter of development begins. The fertilized egg, now called a zygote, starts its journey down the fallopian tube towards the uterus. During this voyage, the zygote undergoes multiple cell divisions, creating a cluster of cells called a blastocyst. This tiny, hollow ball of cells carries the potential for new life.

As the blastocyst reaches the uterus, it must establish a secure connection with the uterine lining. This process is known as implantation. The blastocyst burrows into the endometrial wall, finding a cozy spot to call home for the next nine months. It's a delicate and intricate process that sets the stage for a healthy pregnancy.

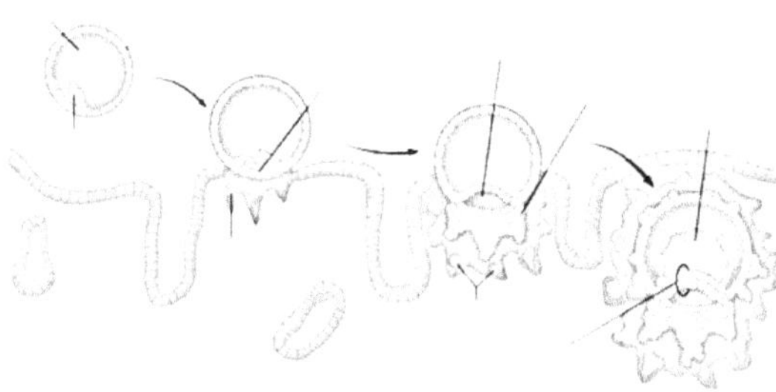

The blastocyst nestles into the uterine lining during the remarkable process of implantation.

1.3   Double Delight: Unveiling the Mysteries of Twin Pregnancies

Twin pregnancies have long captured the imagination and curiosity of humankind. The idea of two souls sharing a womb, destined to embark on life's journey together, is undeniably fascinating. But what exactly sets the stage for these double delights?

Twin pregnancies can be broadly categorized into two types: **Dizygotic** (Fraternal) and **Monozygotic** (Identical). Fraternal twins result from the simultaneous release and fertilization of two separate eggs by two different sperm. In this case, each twin has its unique set of genetic traits, much like any other siblings.

On the other hand, identical twins, a marvel of nature, arise from a single fertilized egg that, at an early stage of development, splits into two embryos. As a result, these twins share identical genetic material and striking physical resemblances. The occurrence of twins is influenced by various factors, including heredity, age, and ethnicity. While fraternal twins may run in families, identical twins are considered a spontaneous phenomenon, occurring at random.

As the twin embryos grow and develop, they may assume different positions in the womb, leading to variations in birth presentations. While some twins are born vertex-vertex (head-first), others might be vertex-breech (head-first and feet-first), or even breech-breech (feet-first).

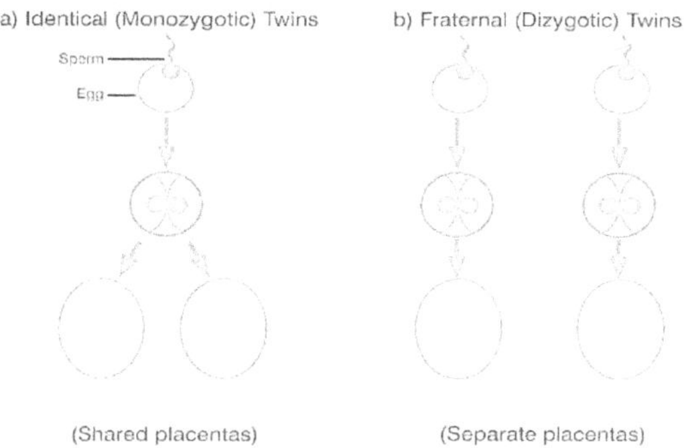

The captivating differences between identical and fraternal twins.

1.4   From Zygote to Embryo: The Remarkable Stages of Early Development

The journey of life begins with a single cell—the zygote. This miraculous cell, formed by the fusion of egg and sperm, carries the genetic blueprint for an entire human being. As it embarks on its path of growth and development, it undergoes an astounding series of transformations. After fertilization, the zygote starts dividing rapidly, forming a cluster of cells that eventually morph into a hollow sphere known as the blastocyst. Within this blastocyst, two distinct cell types emerge—the inner cell mass and the outer layer, each with a unique purpose. The inner cell mass is the origin of the embryo itself—the core of human life-to-be. Meanwhile, the outer layer sets the foundation for the placenta, a remarkable organ that will nourish and protect the developing embryo throughout the pregnancy.

As the embryo continues to grow, it undergoes gastrulation, a process that shapes it into three fundamental layers—the endoderm, mesoderm, and ectoderm. These layers, like the first strokes of an artist's brush, lay the groundwork for the formation of organs, tissues, and the nervous system. Within a few weeks, the embryo transforms into a recognizable human form, complete with a beating heart, limb buds, and the beginnings of facial features. As its tiny heart pumps life-giving blood, the early neural connections form, sparking the foundation of consciousness. The intricate dance of cell division, differentiation, and specialization continues, sculpting the human body with unparalleled precision. The embryo grows larger, and as it enters the fetal stage, it begins to exhibit distinct movements, although the expectant mother may not feel them just yet.

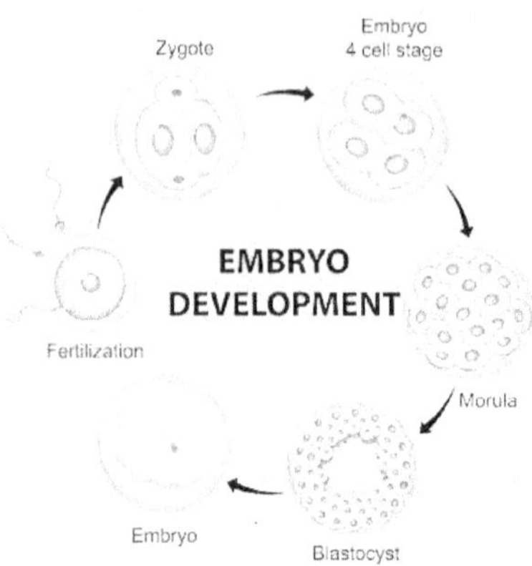

The remarkable stages of early human development from zygote to embryo.

1.5 The Surprising Role of Hormones: Pregnancy's Chemical Symphony

Pregnancy is not only a physical journey but also an intricately orchestrated chemical symphony within the mother's body. Hormones, those powerful messengers secreted by various glands, play a leading role in this symphony, orchestrating a complex dance that supports and nurtures the developing life. The moment of conception sparks a surge in hormone production, signaling the beginning of pregnancy. One of the most critical hormones during this time is human chorionic gonadotropin (hCG). This hormone is what pregnancy tests detect to confirm the presence of a growing life within the woman's womb.

Human chorionic gonadotropin (hCG's) primary function is to maintain the production of progesterone, another vital hormone for pregnancy. Progesterone plays a key role in supporting the thickening of the uterine lining, ensuring that the embryo has a nurturing environment for successful implantation and growth. As the pregnancy progresses, another crucial hormone, estrogen, takes the stage. Produced by the placenta, estrogen plays a multifaceted role. It supports the growth and development of the fetus and prepares the mother's body for labor and breastfeeding.

While estrogen ensures a healthy environment for the growing life, it also influences the maternal body, leading to various changes throughout pregnancy. From the glow of the skin to the relaxation of ligaments in preparation for childbirth, estrogen weaves its magic throughout this transformative journey. Simultaneously, the hormone relaxin works alongside estrogen to relax and widen the ligaments, joints, and tissues in the pelvic region. This allows the mother's body to adapt to the expanding uterus and prepares the birth canal for delivery.

Progesterone, estrogen, and relaxin are just a few of the many hormones choreographing this chemical symphony. Prolactin, for instance, prepares the mother's breasts for lactation, ensuring that she will be able to nourish her baby once born. Oxytocin, often referred to as the "love hormone," takes the center stage during labor, triggering contractions and facilitating the bond between mother and child.

Throughout pregnancy, this harmonious interplay of hormones sustains and nurtures the growing life within. It not only influences the physiological changes in the mother's body but also fosters the emotional bond between her and her unborn child.

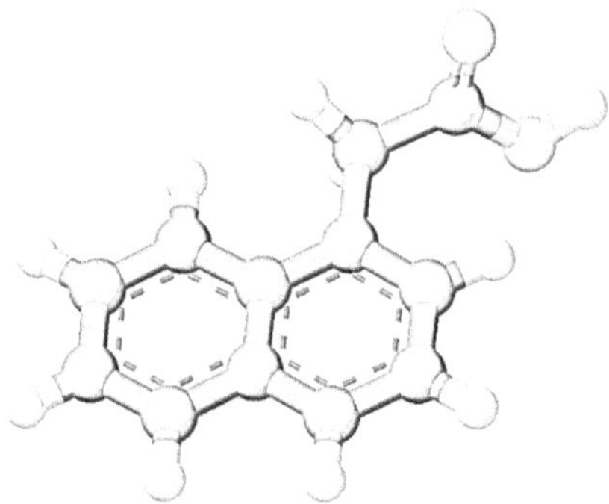

The vital role of hormones in orchestrating pregnancy's chemical symphony.

Chapter 2:
Mind and Body Transformations

2.1 The Pregnancy Glow: Unraveling the Secrets Behind Radiant Skin

Pregnancy is often associated with a radiant glow that seems to emanate from expectant mothers. This phenomenon, aptly named the "pregnancy glow," has captured the curiosity of many. But what exactly causes this transformation in the skin?

During pregnancy, increased blood circulation and hormonal changes play a significant role in creating that radiant complexion. The surge in hormones, particularly estrogen and progesterone, stimulates the sebaceous glands, leading to higher oil production. This natural lubrication can give the skin a smoother and more glowing appearance.

Additionally, increased blood volume and circulation bring more nutrients and oxygen to the skin, enhancing its overall appearance. The "pregnancy glow" is not just a myth; it's a tangible physiological effect of the miraculous changes happening within a woman's body during this unique time.

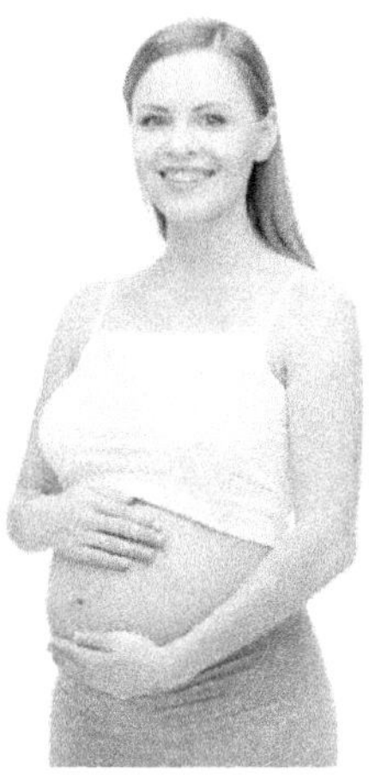

The Pregnancy Glow - Radiant skin due to increased blood circulation and hormonal changes.

2.2 From Head to Toe: How Pregnancy Affects Your Body

Pregnancy brings about a series of transformative changes in a woman's body, both internally and externally. From the moment of conception, the body begins to adapt to accommodate the developing baby.

Internally, the uterus undergoes tremendous expansion to accommodate the growing fetus. As the pregnancy progresses, various organs shift and make space for the baby, which can sometimes lead to discomfort and changes in digestion. Externally, noticeable changes occur in a woman's body as well. The breasts become larger and more sensitive, preparing for milk production. Hormonal changes may lead to darker pigmentation in certain areas, like the nipples and the linea nigra, a dark line that appears on the abdomen. Stretch marks may also develop due to the rapid stretching of the skin.

Weight gain is a natural and essential part of a healthy pregnancy, but it can vary for each woman. Some might gain more weight around the hips and thighs, while others might gain more in the belly region. Embracing these changes and maintaining a healthy lifestyle during pregnancy are vital for the well-being of both the mother and the baby.

2.3 Cravings and Aversions: The Unpredictable Culinary Adventures

One of the most intriguing and well-known aspects of pregnancy is the phenomenon of food cravings and aversions. Many pregnant women experience sudden and intense desires for specific foods, often indulging in unusual combinations or increased quantities. On the flip side, they may also develop strong aversions to foods they once enjoyed.

The root cause of these cravings and aversions is believed to be the fluctuating hormones during pregnancy, primarily the hormones human chorionic gonadotropin (hCG) and estrogen. These hormones can influence the sense of taste and smell, leading to altered food preferences.

Cravings for certain foods may also indicate a deficiency in certain nutrients, prompting the body to seek out those foods as a means of fulfilling its requirements. While it's okay to indulge in cravings occasionally, it's essential to strike a balance and maintain a healthy diet to support the developing baby's needs.

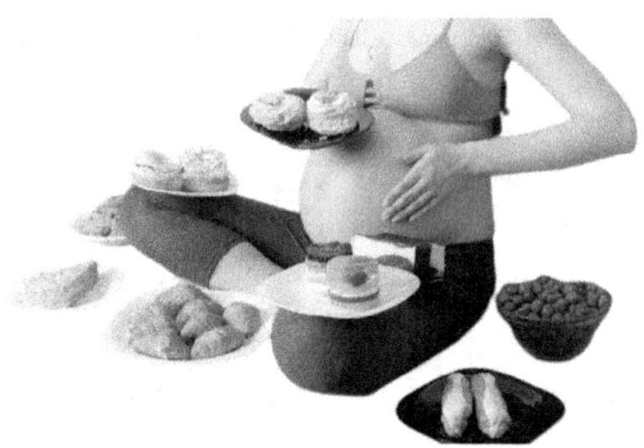

Pregnancy Cravings - Strong desires for specific foods due to hormonal changes.

2.4 Hormonal Rollercoaster: Understanding Emotional Changes

Pregnancy is not just a physical journey; it's an emotional rollercoaster as well. Many pregnant women experience significant mood swings and heightened emotions throughout their pregnancy.

Hormones once again take center stage in influencing these emotional changes. Fluctuations in estrogen and progesterone can impact neurotransmitters in the brain, leading to emotional ups and downs. Additionally, the stress of preparing for parenthood, combined with physical discomfort and fatigue, can further intensify emotional reactions.

It's important for both the expectant mother and her support system to recognize and acknowledge these emotional changes. Providing a supportive and understanding environment can help ease the emotional burden and contribute to a more positive pregnancy experience.

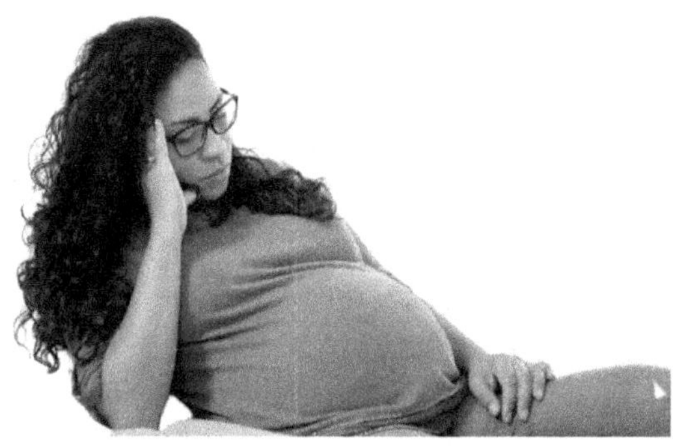

Hormonal Rollercoaster - Emotional changes due to hormonal fluctuations.

2.5 Memory Lapses and "Baby Brain": The Cognitive Impact of Pregnancy

Many pregnant women report experiencing memory lapses, forgetfulness, and a sense of mental fogginess, often referred to as "baby brain." While some may dismiss it as a myth, scientific studies suggest that pregnancy indeed can have cognitive effects.

Hormonal changes, particularly increased levels of estrogen and progesterone, play a significant role in "baby brain." These hormones can impact neurotransmitters in the brain, affecting memory, attention, and cognitive processing. Additionally, the emotional and physical stresses of pregnancy can further contribute to cognitive lapses.

However, it's essential to note that "baby brain" is a temporary condition and does not cause any long-term cognitive impairment. Once the hormones stabilize after childbirth, most women typically return to their pre-pregnancy cognitive abilities.

pregnancy is a time of incredible transformation, both in the body and the mind. Understanding these changes can help expectant mothers embrace and appreciate the unique journey they are embarking on. With proper care, support, and a positive outlook, pregnancy can be a rewarding and fulfilling experience for every mother-to-be.

Chapter 3:

Nourishing Two Lives: The Importance of Diet During Pregnancy

3.1 Building a Strong Foundation: The Essential Nutrients for Expectant Mothers

During pregnancy, a woman's body goes through significant changes, and proper nutrition is crucial for the health and development of both the mother and the growing baby. To ensure a healthy pregnancy journey, it's crucial to focus on essential nutrients that support your baby's growth and keep you in good health. Here are some key nutrients every expectant mother should include in her diet:

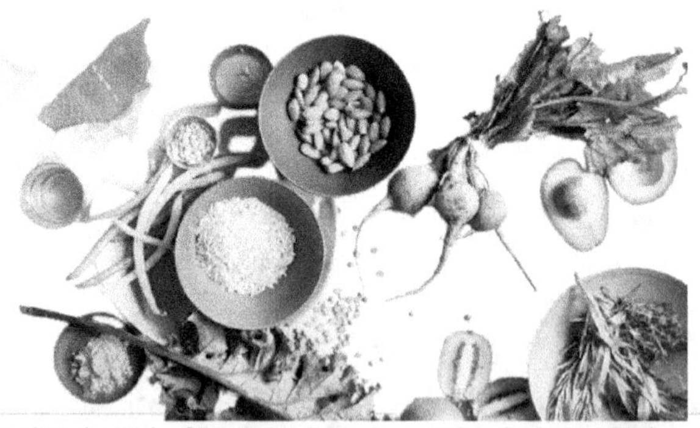

Image of a colorful plate filled with nutrient-rich foods such as leafy greens, fruits, whole grains, and lean proteins.

❖ **Key Nutrients:**

➢ **Folic Acid:** Folic acid helps prevent neural tube defects and supports the baby's brain and spinal cord development.

➢ **Iron:** Adequate iron intake prevents anemia and supports the baby's blood supply.

➢ **Calcium:** Essential for the baby's bone and teeth development.

➢ **Protein:** Supports the growth of tissues and organs in both the mother and baby.

➢ **Omega-3 Fatty Acids:** Important for the baby's brain and eye development.

➢ **Vitamin D:** Supports bone health and immune function.

❖ **Sources of Essential Nutrients:**

➢ **Folate-rich foods:** Leafy greens, legumes, fortified cereals, and citrus fruits.

➢ **Iron-rich foods:** Lean red meats, beans, spinach, and fortified grains.

➢ **Calcium-rich foods:** Dairy products, leafy greens, and fortified plant-based milk.

➢ **Protein-rich foods:** Lean meats, poultry, fish, eggs, tofu, and legumes.

➢ **Omega-3 sources:** Fatty fish (e.g., salmon, mackerel), chia seeds, and walnuts.

➢ **Vitamin D sources:** Sun exposure, fortified dairy products, and supplements.

3.2 Eating for Two: Dispelling Myths and Embracing Healthy Habits

The phrase "eating for two" is often misunderstood, leading to unhealthy eating habits during pregnancy. Let's dispel some common myths and embrace healthy eating habits for expectant mothers.

➢ **Myth #1: I Should Eat Double the Amount.**

Fact: While pregnancy increases caloric needs, it doesn't mean eating twice as much. Extra calories are required, but the focus should be on nutrient-dense foods.

➢ **Myth #2: Indulging in Cravings is Okay.**

Fact: Occasional indulgence is fine, but it's essential to balance cravings with nutrient-rich options. Moderation is key.

➢ **Myth #3: Skipping Meals to Control Weight.**

Fact: Skipping meals deprives the body of essential nutrients. Opt for small, frequent meals to maintain energy levels.

❖ **Healthy Eating Habits:**

  ➢ **Balanced Meals:** Opt for balanced meals that include a variety of fruits, vegetables, whole grains, lean proteins, and healthy fats.

  ➢ **Regular Snacking:** Have small, nutritious snacks throughout the day to maintain steady energy levels and prevent nausea.

  ➢ **Hydration:** Stay well-hydrated by drinking plenty of water, which is essential for the baby's development and overall health.

  ➢ **Limit sugary and processed foods:** These provide empty calories and little nutrition.

  ➢ **Listen to Your Body:** Pay attention to your hunger and fullness cues. Eat when you're hungry and stop when you're satisfied.

  ➢ **Limit Processed Foods:** Minimize the consumption of processed and sugary foods, as they provide empty calories and little nutritional value.

3.3 Food Safety and Pregnancy: A Guide to Making Safe Choices

During pregnancy, a woman's immune system undergoes changes, making her more susceptible to foodborne illnesses. It's essential to make safe food choices to protect both mother and baby.

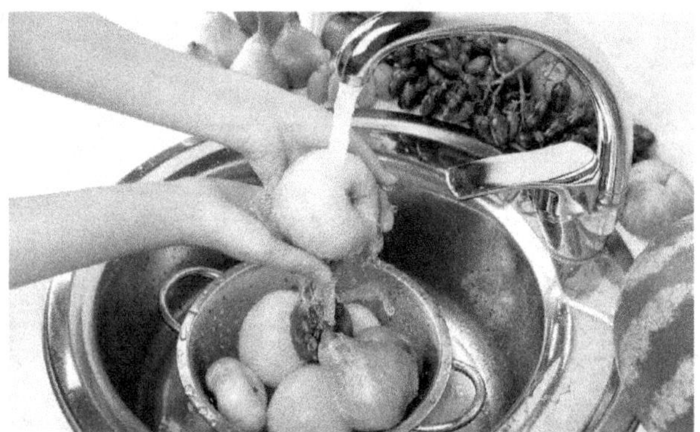

Image depicting proper food handling practices, such as washing vegetables and avoiding raw or undercooked meat.

❖ **Food Safety Tips:**

➢ **Wash hands thoroughly:** Always wash hands before preparing or eating food.

➢ **Avoid certain foods:** Steer clear of raw or undercooked meat, eggs, and fish, as well as unpasteurized dairy products and juices.

➢ **Food Preparation:** Wash fruits and vegetables thoroughly, and practice good hygiene during food preparation.

➢ **Store food properly:** Store perishable foods properly and ensure your refrigerator is set to the right temperature.

➢ **Use separate cutting boards:** Avoid cross-contamination between raw meat and other foods.

➢ **Food Labels:** Pay attention to expiration dates and food labels to make informed choices about the products you consume.

3.4 Managing Weight Gain: Striking a Balance for Mom and Baby

Weight gain during pregnancy is natural and necessary for the baby's growth. However, it's essential to strike a balance and manage weight gain in a healthy way.

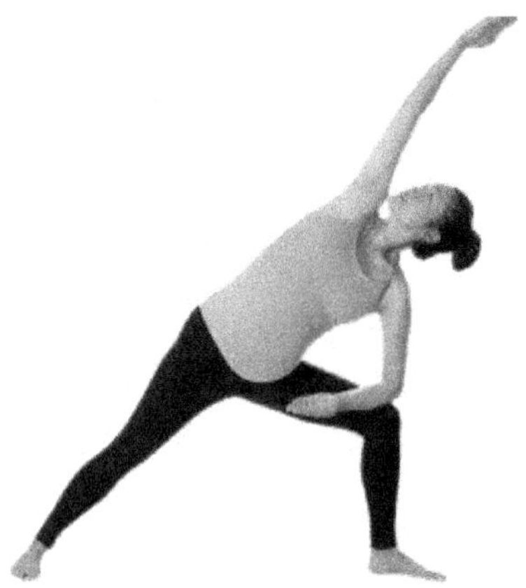

Image of a pregnant woman engaging in safe, pregnancy-friendly exercises, such as prenatal yoga or walking.

❖ **Managing Weight Gain**

Here are some tips:

> **Eat Mindfully:** Focus on nutritious foods and avoid overeating to prevent excessive weight gain.

> **Track weight gain:** Regularly monitor weight with the guidance of a healthcare provider.

> **Focus on nutrition:** Emphasize nutrient-dense foods rather than empty calories.

> **Practice mindfulness:** Listen to hunger cues and eat when genuinely hungry.

> **Stay Physically Active:** Engage in regular, safe exercise as recommended by your healthcare provider.

> **Embrace Body Changes:** Understand that weight gain is a natural part of pregnancy and embrace the changes your body goes through.

> **Avoid Crash Diets:** Never attempt weight loss diets or extreme measures during pregnancy, as they can harm both you and your baby.

3.5 Dealing with Pregnancy Cravings: Satisfying Urges Without Compromising Health

Pregnancy cravings are common and often intensified due to hormonal changes. While it's normal to have cravings, it's essential to manage them in a way that doesn't compromise overall health.

❖ **Tips to Deal with Pregnancy Cravings**

> **Understand the craving:** Sometimes, a craving may indicate a nutrient deficiency. Try to address the underlying need with healthier options.

> **Choose nutritious alternatives:** Opt for healthier versions of cravings, like frozen yogurt instead of ice cream or baked sweet potato fries instead of regular fries.

> **Practice portion control:** Enjoy indulgent treats in moderation.

> **Distract yourself:** Engage in activities to take your mind off cravings, such as going for a walk or spending time with loved ones.

By understanding cravings and making mindful choices, expectant mothers can satisfy their urges while maintaining a healthy and balanced diet.

Chapter 4:

Fascinating Facts about the Growing Bump

4.1 The Marvel of Stretch Marks: Science Behind the Lines

Stretch marks are a common phenomenon during pregnancy that many expectant mothers experience. These reddish, pinkish, or purplish lines on the skin can appear on the belly, breasts, hips, and thighs as the skin stretches to accommodate the growing baby bump. But have you ever wondered what causes these marks?

❖ **Stretch Marks**

Stretch marks, also known as striae gravidarum, occur when the skin is stretched beyond its elastic limits due to rapid weight gain or expansion. During pregnancy, hormonal changes, particularly an increase in cortisol levels, can weaken the skin's collagen and elastin fibers, making it more prone to tearing. As the baby grows, the skin's inability to keep up with the expanding belly leads to the formation of stretch marks.

❖ The Role of Genetics

Genetics also play a significant role in determining who might be more prone to developing stretch marks. If your mother or other close family members experienced them during their pregnancies, there is a higher likelihood that you may develop them too.

❖ Preventing and Minimizing Stretch Marks

While it's difficult to completely prevent stretch marks, there are some steps you can take to minimize their appearance:

- **Stay Hydrated:** Drink plenty of water to keep your skin hydrated and supple.
- **Moisturize:** Applying moisturizers or oils to your belly, breasts, and hips can help improve the skin's elasticity.
- **Maintain a Healthy Diet:** Eating foods rich in vitamins A, C, and E can promote healthy skin.
- **Manage Weight Gain:** Gradual and steady weight gain can reduce the stress on the skin.

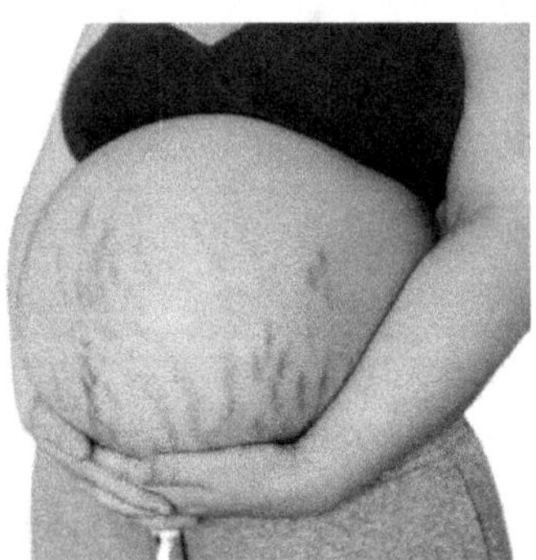

A close-up image of stretch marks on a pregnant belly, showcasing the common occurrence during pregnancy.

4.2 It's Kicking! The Thrilling World of Fetal Movement

One of the most exciting and reassuring moments during pregnancy is feeling your baby's movements for the first time. These tiny flutters and kicks signify the presence of life within you, and they become more pronounced as your baby grows. But what causes these delightful sensations?

❖ When Do You Feel Your Baby Move?

Most women feel their baby's movements between 18 and 25 weeks of pregnancy. However, first-time mothers may not recognize these movements until later, around 25 weeks, as they might mistake them for gas or other bodily sensations initially.

❖ Understanding Fetal Movement

Fetal movement, also known as quickening, occurs as your baby's nervous system develops, and they gain the strength to move their muscles. At first, the movements are gentle and may feel like soft flutters. As the weeks progress, you'll experience more distinct kicks, punches, and rolls as your baby becomes more active.

❖ Bonding with Your Baby

Feeling your baby move is a wonderful opportunity to bond with them even before birth. You can respond to the movements by gently placing your hand on your belly, which may encourage the baby to respond in kind. This interaction creates an emotional connection between you and your little one.

❖ Counting Kicks

In the later stages of pregnancy, healthcare providers often recommend kick counting. This involves monitoring your baby's movements and ensuring they maintain their regular pattern. Any significant decrease in fetal movement might indicate a potential issue, and you should consult your healthcare provider immediately.

4.3 The Mystery of Belly Button Popping Out

As the baby grows and the uterus expands, many pregnant women notice a peculiar change in their belly button—it starts to pop out! This phenomenon is called "umbilical protrusion," and while it may appear unusual, it's entirely normal during pregnancy.

The reason behind this belly button transformation lies in the stretching of the abdominal wall. As the uterus expands, it pushes against the abdominal muscles, causing the belly button, which is essentially a scar from the umbilical cord, to protrude outward.

Not all women experience this change; some may notice their belly buttons becoming flatter or simply remaining unchanged. The extent of the protrusion can vary from person to person and even between pregnancies.

After giving birth, the belly button usually returns to its pre-pregnancy state over time. However, some women may notice that their belly button looks slightly different from before due to the stretching of the skin and tissues during pregnancy.

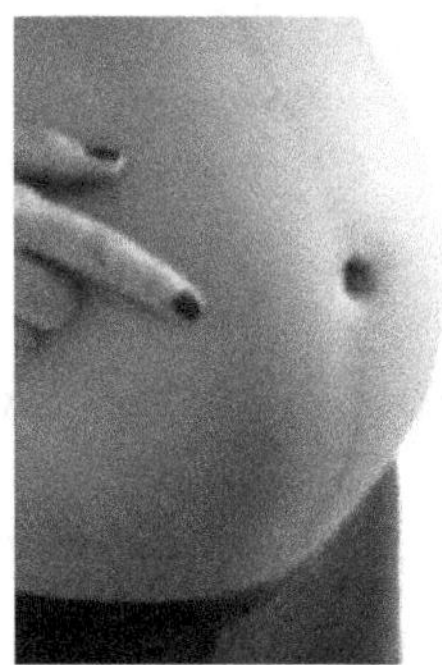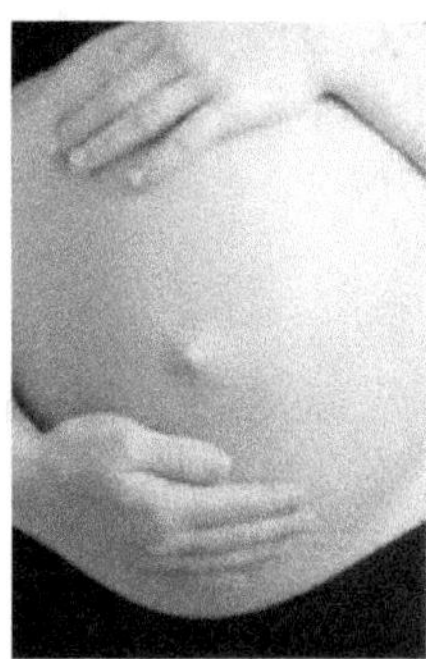

An illustration depicting the transformation of a belly button from an innie to an outie during pregnancy.

4.4 Pregnancy Dreams and Their Symbolism

Pregnancy often brings about a myriad of vivid and sometimes bizarre dreams for expectant mothers. These dreams can range from delightful and soothing to downright strange and frightening. While some women may find these dreams entertaining or unsettling, they are a completely normal part of the journey.

Pregnancy dreams can be influenced by various factors, including hormonal changes, anxieties, and the profound emotional and psychological shifts that occur during this transformative time.

Common themes in pregnancy dreams may include giving birth to animals, losing the baby, or experiencing fantastical adventures.

Psychologists suggest that these dreams often serve as a way for the subconscious mind to process fears, expectations, and hopes related to pregnancy and motherhood. They can also reflect a woman's anxieties about her changing body, her ability to care for the baby, and her transition into motherhood.

Instead of being alarmed by pregnancy dreams, embracing them as a natural part of the experience can be empowering. Many cultures believe that dreams during pregnancy carry special meaning and can offer insights into the upcoming chapter of life. Keeping a dream journal can help mothers explore their emotions and gain a deeper understanding of their feelings and concerns.

4.5 Carrying High or Low: Debunking Belly Position Myths

Throughout pregnancy, friends, family, and even strangers might speculate about whether a woman is carrying the baby "high" or "low" based on the shape of her baby bump. According to popular folklore, carrying high indicates the baby is a girl, while carrying low means it's a boy. However, there is no scientific evidence to support these claims.

The position of the baby bump primarily depends on the individual's body shape, abdominal muscles, and the baby's position within the uterus. Factors like the mother's muscle tone, the number of previous pregnancies, and the baby's size can influence the bump's appearance.

If the baby is positioned higher in the uterus, the bump may appear to be higher. On the other hand, if the baby is positioned lower, the bump might look lower and closer to the pelvic region.

It's important to remember that the position of the baby bump doesn't reveal the baby's gender. The only accurate way to determine the baby's sex is through medical tests like ultrasound or genetic testing. Pregnancy is a remarkable journey filled with numerous unique and intriguing aspects. Understanding the science behind all this phenomenon contribute to a deeper appreciation of the miraculous process of bringing new life into the world.

Chapter 5:

Navigating the Ups and Downs of Pregnancy

5.1 Morning Sickness: Causes, Remedies, and Myths

Morning sickness, despite its name, can occur at any time of the day. It is experienced by the majority of pregnant women, and while it is not entirely understood, hormonal changes and an increase in human chorionic gonadotropin (hCG) levels are believed to play a role. Here are some intriguing facts and helpful tips to cope with morning sickness:

❖ **Causes of Morning Sickness:**

➤ Hormonal fluctuations, particularly increased hCG levels.

➤ Enhanced sensitivity to smells and tastes.

➤ Changes in digestion and metabolism.

➤ Emotional and psychological factors.

❖ Remedies for Morning Sickness:

- Eat small, frequent meals to avoid an empty stomach.
- Stay hydrated by drinking plenty of water.
- Avoid spicy, greasy, and strong-smelling foods.
- Ginger has been found to alleviate nausea, try ginger tea or ginger candies.
- Get plenty of rest and manage stress levels.

❖ Morning Sickness Myths

a)   **Myth:** Only happens in the morning.

Reality: Morning sickness can occur at any time of the day.

b)   **Myth:** Indicates the baby's gender.

Reality: Morning sickness is not a reliable predictor of the baby's gender.

c)   **Myth:** Severe morning sickness means a healthier pregnancy.

Reality: The severity of morning sickness doesn't necessarily indicate the health of the pregnancy.

Remember, morning sickness is usually temporary and tends to subside by the second trimester. If you're experiencing excessive vomiting and are unable to keep food or liquids down, consult your healthcare provider.

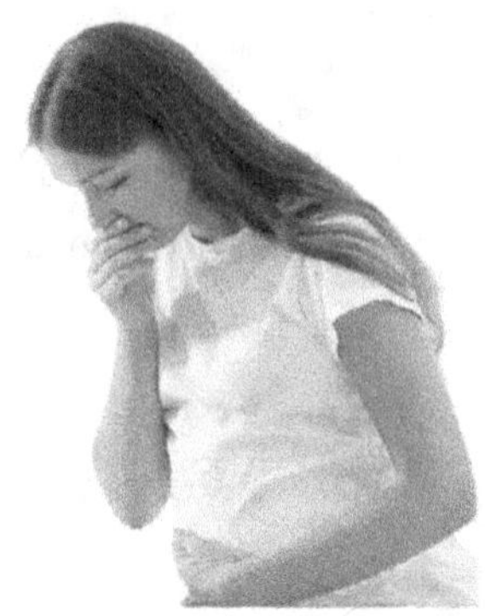

Morning sickness is a common pregnancy symptom that can affect women during the first trimester.

4.2 The Second Trimester: Golden Period of Pregnancy

The second trimester is a beautiful phase for most expectant mothers. Often considered the "golden period," it spans from weeks 13 to 27 of pregnancy. Here's what makes this phase so special and some essential things to keep in mind:

❖ **Feeling Better**

> ➤ Morning sickness typically subsides, and energy levels improve.
> ➤ The risk of miscarriage decreases significantly.
> ➤ Most women experience an increase in libido.

❖ **Baby Bump and Bonding:**

> ➤ The baby bump becomes more noticeable, bringing joy and excitement.
> ➤ You may start feeling your baby's movements (quickening), creating a strong bond.

❖ **Ultrasound and Gender Reveal**

> ➤ Many women have their first ultrasound during this trimester, allowing them to see their baby.
> ➤ Around week 20, you can often find out the baby's gender if you choose to.

❖ **Self-Care and Preparing for Birth:**

> Engage in gentle exercises like prenatal yoga to stay active and relieve discomfort.

> Consider attending childbirth classes to prepare for labor and delivery.

> Start thinking about baby names and nursery decoration.

However, remember that every pregnancy is unique, and some discomforts like back pain and constipation may still persist. Stay in touch with your healthcare provider and enjoy this wonderful phase of pregnancy.

4.3 Heartburn and Indigestion: Taming the Fire Within

As the uterus expands, it puts pressure on the stomach, leading to heartburn and indigestion. Hormonal changes that relax the lower esophageal sphincter (LES) can also contribute to this uncomfortable issue. Here's how you can tame the fire within:

❖ **Dietary Adjustments:**

> Eat smaller, more frequent meals to prevent overloading your stomach.

> Avoid spicy, acidic, and fatty foods that can trigger heartburn.

> Opt for high-fiber foods to aid digestion and avoid constipation.

❖ **Eating Habits:**

> Avoid lying down immediately after eating; try to stay upright for some time.

> Use extra pillows while sleeping to keep your upper body elevated.

❖ **Natural Remedies:**

> Sip on chamomile or peppermint tea to soothe the digestive system.

> A tablespoon of apple cider vinegar in water may help neutralize stomach acid.

❖ **Consult Your Healthcare Provider**

If heartburn becomes severe or persistent, consult your healthcare provider. They may recommend safe antacids or other suitable remedies to provide relief.

❖

4.4 Sleeping Woes: Finding Comfort in the Land of Nod

As your belly grows, finding a comfortable sleeping position can be quite challenging. Additionally, hormonal changes, frequent trips to the bathroom, and anxiety may interfere with your sleep. Here are some tips to help you find comfort in the land of nod:

❖ **Sleeping Positions:**
   ➢ Sleep on your side, preferably the left side, to improve blood circulation and nutrient flow to the baby.
   ➢ Use pillows to support your belly, back, and knees for added comfort.

❖ **Nighttime Routine:**
   ➢ Establish a calming bedtime routine to signal your body that it's time to wind down.
   ➢ Limit fluids a few hours before bedtime to reduce nighttime bathroom visits.

❖ **Relaxation Techniques:**
   ➢ Practice deep breathing or prenatal yoga to relax before bedtime.
   ➢ Consider using pregnancy-safe essential oils like lavender for relaxation.

❖ **Create a Relaxing Environment**
   ➢ Keep the bedroom cool, dark, and quiet for better sleep quality.
   ➢ Use a white noise machine if outside sounds disturb your sleep.

4.5 The Joys and Challenges of the Third Trimester

The third trimester is the final stretch of pregnancy, filled with both joys and challenges. Here's what you can expect during this phase:

❖ **Baby's Growth and Movement:**
   ➢ Your baby is rapidly growing, gaining weight, and developing vital organs.
   ➢ Movements may become more frequent and stronger as your baby has less space to move around.

❖ **Physical Discomforts:**

> ➤ Backaches, swollen feet, and frequent urination may become more pronounced.

> ➤ Braxton Hicks contractions may occur as your body prepares for labor.

❖ **Preparation for Birth:**

> ➤ Attend prenatal classes to learn about childbirth and postpartum care.

> ➤ Pack your hospital bag with essentials for the delivery.

Nesting Instinct:

- Many expectant mothers experience a strong urge to organize and prepare their home for the baby's arrival.

Emotional Roller Coaster:

- Hormonal fluctuations and the anticipation of parenthood can lead to mixed emotions.

Chapter 6:

Unveiling Gender and Genetic Surprises

6.1 From Pink to Blue: Exploring the Science of Gender Prediction

The moment parents-to-be find out the gender of their baby is often filled with excitement and anticipation. Traditionally, baby girls were associated with the color pink, and baby boys with the color blue. However, in today's world, gender reveals have become more creative and personalized. Let's explore the fascinating history behind these gender associations and how modern parents are embracing new ways to celebrate this exciting news.

❖ Pink and Blue Gender Associations

The pink-for-girls and blue-for-boys tradition is relatively recent in history, dating back to the early 20th century. Before that, pastel colors, including pink and blue, were often used interchangeably for both genders. It wasn't until the 1940s that manufacturers and marketers began promoting gender-specific colors. However, these associations have evolved over time, with many parents today choosing gender-neutral colors or even opting not to reveal the gender until birth.

❖ Modern Gender Reveals

Gender reveals have become a creative trend, with parents coming up with innovative ways to share the news with family and friends. From confetti-filled balloons to cutting into a cake to reveal the color inside, the possibilities are endless. Remember, the most important thing is to celebrate the upcoming arrival of your little one, regardless of their gender.

6.2 Genetic Inheritance: Traits Passed Down to Your Baby

Genetic inheritance plays a significant role in determining the characteristics and traits your baby will possess. The study of heredity has fascinated scientists for centuries, and today, we have a better understanding of how genes are passed down from parents to their offspring.

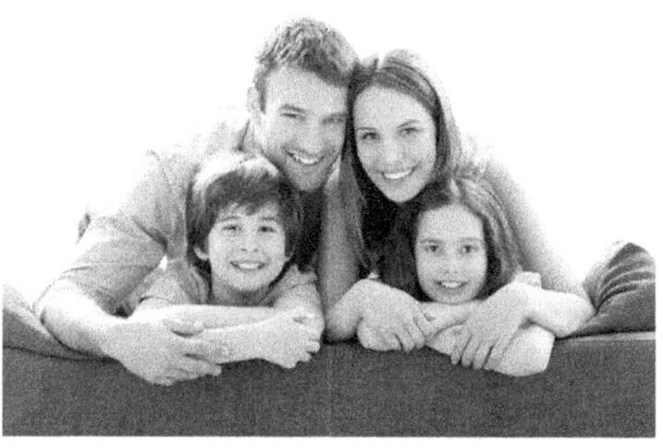

Discovering the remarkable inheritance of traits from one generation to the next.

❖ Dominant and Recessive Traits

Genes come in pairs, with one inherited from each parent. Some genes are dominant, meaning their traits will be expressed even if only one copy is present, while others are recessive, requiring both copies to be present for the trait to show up. For example, if both parents have brown eyes (a dominant trait), their child is likely to have brown eyes as well. However, if both parents carry a recessive gene for blue eyes, their child may inherit blue eyes instead.

❖ Genetic Diversity

Each person's genetic makeup is incredibly diverse, resulting in a wide range of physical features, personality traits, and susceptibilities to certain conditions. Embrace the uniqueness of your baby's genetic inheritance, knowing that their individuality is a beautiful blend of both maternal and paternal genes.

6.3 Old Wives' Tales: Fun Predictors of Baby's Gender

Throughout history, people have relied on various folklore and old wives' tales to predict a baby's gender before the advent of modern technology. While these methods may not have a scientific basis, they can be entertaining and add an element of fun to the pregnancy journey.

Some popular old wives' tales include:

➤ **The Shape of the Bump:** One popular belief suggests that carrying the baby high indicates a girl, while a low bump indicates a boy.

- ➤ **Cravings:** Some say that craving sweets indicates a girl, while cravings for salty or savory foods signal a boy.
- ➤ **Morning Sickness:** The severity of morning sickness is believed by some to be an indicator of baby gender, with more intense sickness pointing to a girl.
- ➤ **Heart Rate:** According to this tale, a higher fetal heart rate indicates a girl, while a lower heart rate suggests a boy.
- ➤ **Chinese Gender Calendar:** This ancient calendar, based on the mother's age at conception and the month of conception, predicts the baby's gender.

Remember, these tales are merely for amusement, and the only surefire way to know your baby's gender is through medical technology like ultrasounds or genetic testing.

6.4 Genetic Testing: Insights into Your Baby's Health

Advancements in medical science have brought us genetic testing, a valuable tool that provides insights into the health and development of your baby during pregnancy. Genetic testing can help identify potential genetic conditions, giving parents an opportunity to prepare and make informed decisions.

Let's explore the different types of genetic tests available and how they contribute to a healthier start for your little one.

❖ **Types of Genetic Tests:**

- ➤ **Carrier Screening:** This test assesses if parents carry certain genetic conditions that could be passed on to their children. It is particularly useful for couples with a family history of genetic disorders.
- ➤ **Non-Invasive Prenatal Testing (NIPT):** NIPT analyzes the baby's DNA present in the mother's blood to screen for chromosomal abnormalities, such as Down syndrome.
- ➤ **Amniocentesis:** In this test, a small sample of amniotic fluid is collected to analyze the baby's chromosomes, providing information about potential genetic conditions.
- ➤ **Chorionic Villus Sampling (CVS):** CVS involves taking a sample of placental tissue to examine the baby's chromosomes and identify any genetic issues.

❖ Empowerment Through Knowledge

Genetic testing offers parents valuable information about their baby's health, allowing them to plan for potential challenges and seek appropriate medical care. Discussing the results with healthcare professionals can help parents understand the implications and make well-informed decisions.

6.5 Surprise, Surprise! Unveiling Unexpected Genetic Conditions

Sometimes, despite all the preparation and testing, unexpected genetic conditions may be revealed after the baby's birth. While this can be challenging news for parents, remember that support and resources are available to help you navigate this journey. Here are how parents can navigate this journey with love, support, and the help of medical professionals.

❖ Receiving the News

Learning that your baby has an unexpected genetic condition can be overwhelming and emotional. It's essential to give yourself time to process the information and seek support from your loved ones and healthcare team.

❖ Accessing Support and Resources

Numerous support groups and resources are available for parents navigating the complexities of raising a child with a genetic condition. Connecting with others who have experienced similar situations can provide comfort, advice, and a sense of community.

❖ Medical Care and Early Interventions

Working closely with healthcare professionals, early interventions can be planned to provide the best possible care for your baby. Early treatment and therapies can significantly improve the child's quality of life and development.

❖ Embracing Parenthood

Parenting a child with a genetic condition can be both challenging and rewarding. Embrace the journey, celebrate your child's milestones, and focus on creating a loving and supportive environment where they can thrive.

Chapter 7:
Preparing for Labor and Beyond

7.1 Braxton Hicks Contractions: False Alarms and Practice Runs

As your due date approaches, you may experience Braxton Hicks contractions. These contractions are not true labor contractions, but rather, they are practice runs that your uterus undergoes in preparation for the real deal. Understanding Braxton Hicks contractions can help ease any unnecessary anxiety during your pregnancy journey.

❖ What are Braxton Hicks Contractions?

Braxton Hicks contractions are intermittent, irregular contractions of the uterus that can begin as early as the second trimester. Unlike true labor contractions, they do not dilate the cervix or lead to childbirth. Instead, they are the body's way of "practicing" for labor, helping to tone and strengthen the uterine muscles.

❖ Differentiating Braxton Hicks from Real Contractions

It is essential to recognize the difference between Braxton Hicks and true labor contractions. Braxton Hicks contractions tend to be milder and more sporadic than genuine labor contractions. They often stop when you change positions, hydrate, or rest. True labor contractions, on the other hand, become progressively more intense, frequent, and regular.

❖ How to Recognize Braxton Hicks Contractions

> **Timing:** Braxton Hicks Contractions tend to be irregular and sporadic, coming and going without a consistent pattern.

> **Pain Level:** They are usually painless or mildly uncomfortable, feeling more like a tightening sensation in your abdomen.

> **Activity and Rest:** These contractions may be more noticeable after physical activity and can often subside with rest or a change in position.

➢ **Lack of Progression:** Unlike true labor contractions, Braxton Hicks Contractions do not intensify over time or cause cervical dilation.

❖ **Managing Braxton Hicks Contractions**

While Braxton Hicks Contractions are a normal part of pregnancy, they may become bothersome for some women. Here are some tips to ease any discomfort:

➢ **Stay Hydrated:** Dehydration can sometimes trigger Braxton Hicks Contractions, so make sure you drink plenty of water.

➢ **Change Positions:** If you feel the contractions becoming uncomfortable, try changing positions or lying down to see if they subside.

➢ **Take Deep Breaths:** Practicing deep breathing techniques can help you relax and reduce the intensity of the contractions.

❖ **When to Seek Medical Attention**

In most cases, Braxton Hicks Contractions are harmless and part of a normal pregnancy. However, if you experience any of the following symptoms, it's essential to contact your healthcare provider:

➢ **Severe Pain:** If the contractions become painful and are accompanied by lower back pain or pressure, it may be a sign of preterm labor.

➢ **Increased Frequency:** If you notice a sudden increase in the frequency of contractions, especially before 37 weeks, consult your doctor.

➢ **Watery Discharge:** Any leaking or gushing of fluid may indicate that your water has broken, and you should seek medical attention immediately.

Remember, every pregnancy is different, so if you're ever unsure or concerned about any symptoms, it's best to reach out to your healthcare provider.

7.2 The Art of Breathing: Techniques for Labor and Delivery

The birthing process can be intense, and having effective breathing techniques can significantly impact your experience during labor and delivery. Learning the art of breathing can empower you to cope with pain, reduce stress, and maintain focus throughout this miraculous journey.

❖ The Power of Deep Breathing

Deep breathing is the foundation of effective birthing techniques. It helps you relax, oxygenates your body, and encourages the release of endorphins, natural pain-relieving hormones.

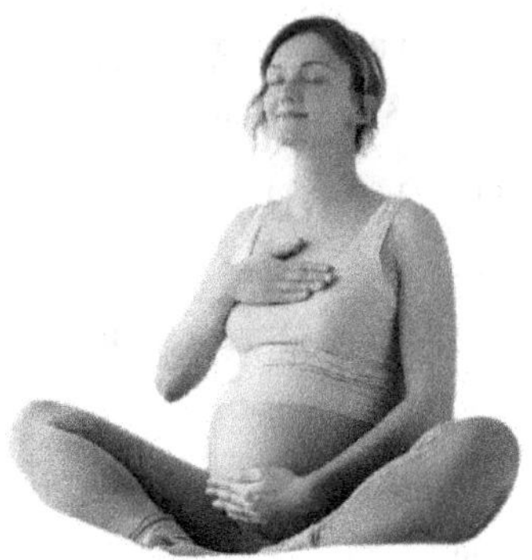

Proper breathing techniques can help manage pain and stress during labor and delivery.

❖ Different Breathing Techniques

> **Slow Belly Breaths:** Inhale deeply through your nose, feeling your belly rise like a balloon. Exhale slowly through your mouth, imagining you are blowing out a candle. This technique helps you stay calm and centered.

> **Rhythmic Breathing:** Establish a steady rhythm of breathing in and out. For example, inhale for a count of four and exhale for a count of four. This technique provides focus during contractions.

> **Patterned Breathing:** During contractions, follow a specific breathing pattern, such as "hee-hee-hoo" or "peace-release." These patterns can distract from pain and keep you focused.

❖ The Role of a Supportive Partner

Having a supportive partner during labor is invaluable. Encourage your partner to practice these breathing techniques with you during pregnancy. They can remind you to breathe properly during labor and provide a comforting presence.

Breathing techniques are essential tools for managing the challenges of labor and delivery. Practicing these techniques during pregnancy will help you develop confidence in your ability to handle whatever comes your way on the day of your baby's arrival.

7.3 Baby's First Cry: Why It's a Magical Sound

The moment a baby enters the world, one of the most heartwarming sounds you'll hear is their first cry. This magical sound signifies more than just communication; it plays a vital role in the baby's transition from the womb to the outside world.

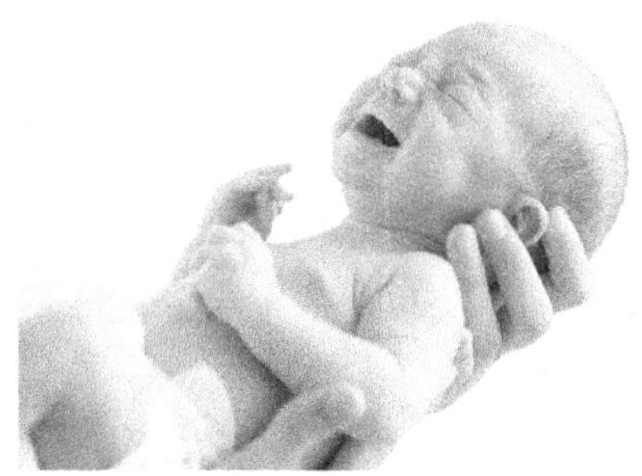

A baby's first cry is an important milestone and a sign of a healthy respiratory system.

❖ **Importance of Baby's First Cry**

  ➢ **Clearing Air Passages:** During pregnancy, the baby's lungs are filled with fluid. The first cry helps expel this fluid and replace it with air, clearing the airways for proper breathing.

  ➢ **Indicating Lung Readiness:** A robust cry indicates that the baby's lungs are mature and ready for independent breathing. This is a reassuring sign of the baby's overall health.

  ➢ **Establishing Respiration:** Crying stimulates the respiratory system, initiating the exchange of oxygen and carbon dioxide in the lungs, promoting a self-sustained breathing pattern.

  ➢ **Sign of Vigor:** A strong cry shows that the baby is alert, responsive, and has a healthy nervous system.

❖ **The Emotional Impact**

Beyond its physiological significance, a baby's first cry evokes powerful emotions in parents and medical professionals. It symbolizes the beginning of a new life journey, marking the start of the parent-child bond.

7.4 The Hormonal Orchestra: The Role of Oxytocin in Labor

Oxytocin, often referred to as the "love hormone" or "bonding hormone," is a remarkable chemical messenger that plays a central role in labor, childbirth, and the formation of maternal-infant attachment.

❖ The Role of Oxytocin in Labor

> **Uterine Contractions:** Oxytocin stimulates uterine contractions during labor. It helps the uterus to contract and progress toward delivery, assisting in the dilation and effacement of the cervix.

> **Pain Management:** This hormone also has a pain-relieving effect during labor. As oxytocin levels rise, the body's endorphins increase, helping the mother cope with pain and stress.

> **Maternal Bonding:** Oxytocin fosters the emotional bond between the mother and her newborn. It enhances feelings of love, trust, and affection, promoting mother-infant attachment.

> **Breastfeeding:** Oxytocin is vital for successful breastfeeding. It triggers the let-down reflex, allowing milk to flow from the breasts, and contributes to the emotional connection between mother and baby during nursing.

❖ Promoting Oxytocin Release

Several factors can enhance oxytocin release during labor and beyond:

- Skin-to-skin contact with the baby immediately after birth.
- Frequent breastfeeding and kangaroo care (skin-to-skin contact) in the early postpartum period.
- A calm and supportive birthing environment.
- Positive and reassuring interactions with caregivers and partners.

7.5 Packing Your Hospital Bag: Essentials and Personal Touches

As your due date draws near, it's essential to have your hospital bag ready. Preparing a well-thought-out hospital bag ensures that you have everything you need to make your labor and postpartum experience as comfortable and stress-free as possible. Let's take a look at some essentials and personal touches to consider when packing your hospital bag.

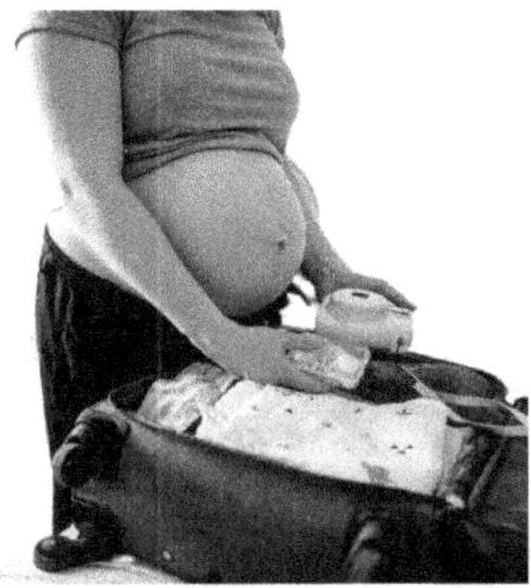

Packing a well-prepared hospital bag can help ensure a smoother and more comfortable labor experience

❖ **Essentials for Labor and Delivery**

➢ **Comfortable Clothing:** Pack loose, comfortable clothing for labor, such as a comfortable nightgown or a loose-fitting, button-down shirt. Don't forget extra underwear and socks.

➢ **Toiletries:** Bring your toothbrush, toothpaste, shampoo, conditioner, body wash, and any other personal toiletries you prefer.

➢ **Snacks and Drinks:** Labor can be a lengthy process, so pack some snacks and drinks to keep your energy up.

➢ **Phone and Charger:** You'll want to stay connected and capture precious moments, so make sure your phone is fully charged and pack a charger.

➢ **Hospital Documents and Insurance:** Organize your identification, hospital documents, and insurance information in a folder for easy access. If you have a birth plan, bring a copy to discuss with your healthcare provider.

➢ **Comfort Items:** Consider bringing items that bring you comfort, like a favorite pillow or a cozy blanket.

❖ **Personal Touches: Making Your Space Feel Like Home**

> - **Family Photos:** Bring some framed photos of your loved ones to personalize your hospital room.
> - **Music or Audiobooks:** Create a playlist of your favorite songs or calming music, or download some audiobooks to help you relax during labor.
> - **Essential Oils:** Some women find aromatherapy helpful during labor. Bring some essential oils and a diffuser if you enjoy this practice.
> - **Journal:** Pack a journal to jot down your thoughts and feelings during this momentous occasion.
> - **Baby Book:** If you have a baby book, bring it along so you can record your baby's first moments.

❖ **For the Postpartum Period**

> - **Comfortable Clothing:** Pack loose, comfortable clothing for the postpartum period, including nursing bras and maternity underwear.
> - **Toiletries:** Make sure to have supplies for postpartum care, such as maternity pads, nipple cream, and a peri bottle.
> - **Going-Home Outfit:** Choose a comfortable outfit for you and your baby to wear when leaving the hospital.
> - **Baby Essentials:** Pack essentials for your newborn, including diapers, wipes, and a swaddle blanket.
> - **Car Seat:** Have your car seat properly installed in your vehicle for bringing your baby home safely.

Remember that every woman's needs and preferences are unique, so customize your hospital bag based on what will make you feel most comfortable and supported during this special time.

Chapter 8:

Postpartum Surprises and Joys

Congratulations on your new bundle of joy! Welcoming a newborn into your life is an incredible journey filled with both surprises and joys. In this chapter, we will explore the challenges and rewards of the postpartum period, providing valuable insights and tips to help you navigate this beautiful phase of life.

8.1 The Fourth Trimester: Adjusting to Life with a Newborn

The Fourth Trimester is a critical time when your baby is adjusting to life outside the womb and getting used to the new world around them. It usually lasts from birth to around three months of age. During this time, parents may encounter various surprises and challenges:

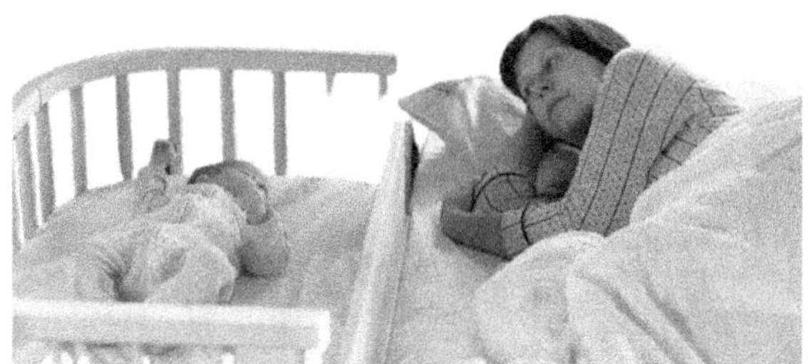

Image of a peaceful sleeping newborn baby in a crib

- ➤ **Sleep patterns:** Newborns have erratic sleep patterns, waking up multiple times during the night for feeding and comfort. It can be exhausting for parents, but rest assured, this phase is temporary.
- ➤ **Feeding cues:** Understanding your baby's hunger cues is essential. Crying isn't the only indication of hunger; rooting, sucking on fists, and smacking lips can also signal hunger.

➢ **Developmental milestones:** Despite being very young, babies begin to show signs of development. They may start to smile, coo, and grasp objects.

➢ **Bonding:** Building a strong bond with your baby during the Fourth Trimester is vital. Skin-to-skin contact, gentle touch, and soothing sounds help strengthen the parent-child relationship.

➢ **Self-care:** It's essential to take care of yourself during this time of adjustment. Rest when your baby sleeps, ask for help from friends or family, and don't hesitate to seek professional support if needed.

Remember, every baby is unique, and there's no one-size-fits-all approach to parenting during the Fourth Trimester. Be patient with yourself and your baby, and cherish the small joys of this precious time.

8.2 Baby Blues or Postpartum Depression: Navigating Emotional Changes

After childbirth, many new mothers experience a range of emotions, often referred to as the "baby blues." These feelings can include mood swings, sadness, irritability, and anxiety. The baby blues are a common and usually short-lived phenomenon, typically lasting for a few days to a couple of weeks.

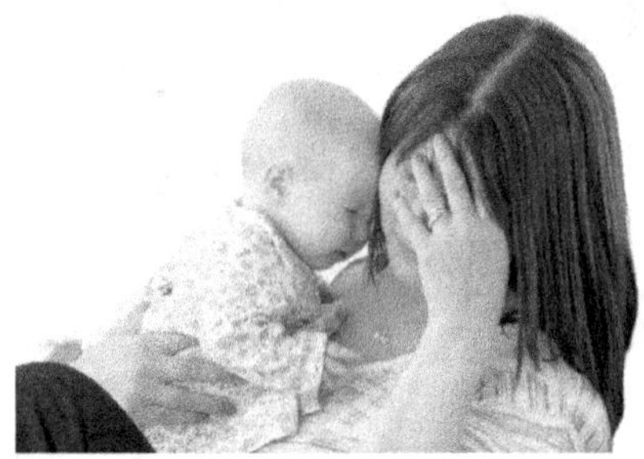

Understanding the difference between the "baby blues" and postpartum depression is crucial in supporting new moms emotionally.

However, for some women, these emotional changes can become more severe and prolonged, leading to postpartum depression (PPD). PPD is a serious condition that affects about 1 in 10 new mothers. It's crucial to recognize the signs of postpartum depression and seek help if needed:

- ➤ Persistent feelings of sadness, hopelessness, or worthlessness
- ➤ Loss of interest or pleasure in activities once enjoyed
- ➤ Changes in appetite and sleep patterns
- ➤ Difficulty bonding with the baby
- ➤ Intense irritability and anger
- ➤ Thoughts of self-harm or harming the baby

If you or someone you know is experiencing these symptoms, it's essential to reach out for support. Speak to your healthcare provider, a therapist, or a support group specializing in postpartum mental health. Remember, seeking help is a sign of strength, and early intervention can lead to a more positive outcome.

8.3 The Truth About Baby Weight: Losing and Loving Your Postpartum Body

After giving birth, many new mothers are eager to shed the baby weight and return to their pre-pregnancy shape. However, it's essential to approach postpartum weight loss with patience and self-compassion. Here are some truths about postpartum weight and body acceptance:

- **Everybody is different:** Each woman's postpartum journey is unique. Some may lose weight quickly, while others may take more time. Comparing your progress to others can be discouraging, so focus on your own health and well-being.
- **Nourishment is essential:** Instead of going on restrictive diets, focus on nourishing your body with healthy and balanced meals. This approach benefits both you and your baby if you're breastfeeding.
- **Gentle exercises:** Engage in gentle exercises, such as walking, yoga, or postpartum-specific workouts, to rebuild strength and stamina gradually.
- **Celebrate small victories:** Celebrate every achievement, no matter how small. Whether it's fitting into your favorite jeans or achieving a fitness milestone, acknowledge your progress.
- **Love your body:** Your body has gone through incredible changes to bring new life into the world. Embrace these changes and appreciate the beauty of your postpartum body.

Remember that weight loss should never be rushed, and it's essential to prioritize your physical and emotional well-being over societal pressures.

8.4 Breastfeeding Mysteries: From Supply to Latching

Breastfeeding is a beautiful and natural way to nourish your baby, but it can also be a mysterious and challenging journey. Here are some common breastfeeding mysteries and how to navigate them:

- ➢ **Milk supply:** Understanding your baby's feeding cues and nursing on demand helps establish a healthy milk supply. Remember, breasts may not feel full, but babies can still get enough milk.
- ➢ **Latching:** A proper latch is crucial for effective breastfeeding and preventing discomfort for both mom and baby. Seek guidance from a lactation consultant if you encounter difficulties with latching.
- ➢ **Cluster feeding:** Cluster feeding, where your baby wants to nurse frequently for short periods, is entirely normal, especially during growth spurts. It helps boost milk supply and meet your baby's developmental needs.
- ➢ **Breast care:** Taking care of your breasts is essential during breastfeeding. Use lanolin cream to soothe sore nipples and change nursing pads frequently to prevent infection.
- ➢ **Pumping and storing:** If you plan to pump and store breast milk, make sure to follow proper hygiene and storage guidelines. Invest in a high-quality breast pump for efficient milk expression.

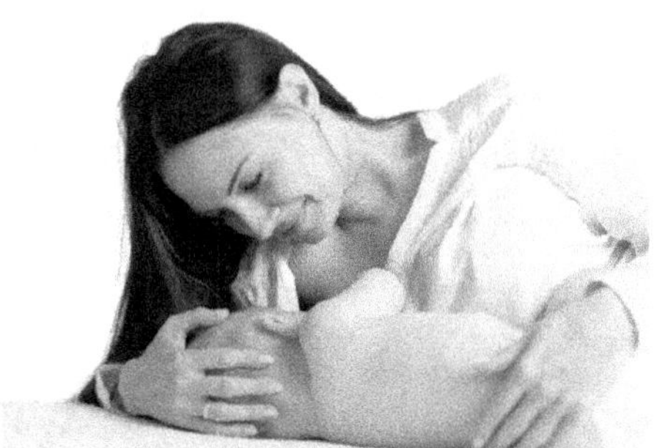

Image of a mother breastfeeding her baby with a peaceful expression

8.5 Sleepless Nights and Sweet Smiles: The Rewards of Parenthood

Parenthood is a beautiful and transformative journey, filled with surprises and joys that await new parents. In this section, we will explore the mixed emotions of sleepless nights and the heartwarming rewards of witnessing your baby's first sweet smiles. These moments, though challenging, are what make the experience of parenthood so special and unforgettable.

❖ Sleepless Nights: Navigating Parenthood's Toughest Challenge

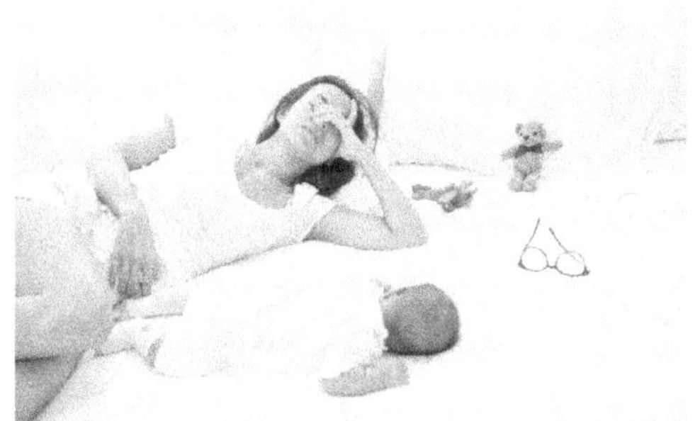

Becoming a parent is a rollercoaster of emotions, and sleepless nights are often the most challenging aspect. As your baby adjusts to their new environment, their sleep patterns may be unpredictable, leading to disrupted nights for you as parents. It's essential to remember that this phase is temporary and part of your baby's natural development. Here are some helpful tips to navigate these sleepless nights:

Create a consistent bedtime routine: Establishing a calming routine before bedtime can signal to your baby that it's time to sleep, helping them settle more easily.

Share the nighttime responsibilities: If possible, take turns with your partner for nighttime feedings and diaper changes, providing each other with much-needed rest.

Embrace napping: Rest whenever your baby naps during the day to recharge and regain energy.

Seek support: Reach out to friends, family, or support groups to share experiences and gain valuable advice.

The Science of Baby Smiles: Unraveling the Magic

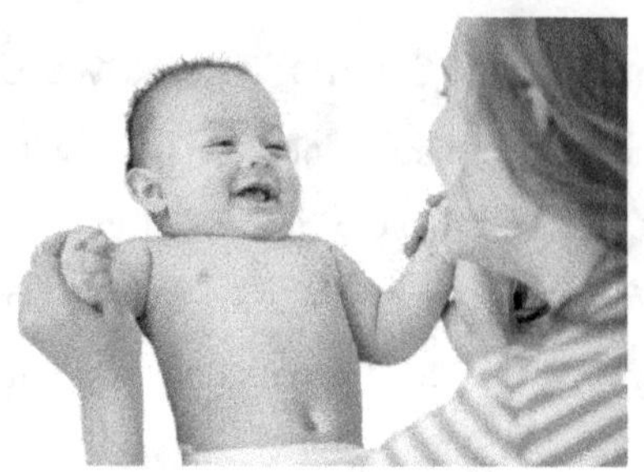

One of the most heartwarming rewards of parenthood is witnessing your baby's first smile. These little gestures are more than just adorable; they signify essential milestones in your baby's development. The science behind baby smiles is fascinating:

- ➤ **Reflexive Smiles:** In their early weeks, babies may exhibit reflexive smiles, which are spontaneous and not a reaction to external stimuli. These usually occur during sleep or after feeding.
- ➤ **Social Smiles:** At around 6 to 8 weeks, babies begin to smile in response to stimuli, such as their parents' voices or faces. This marks the beginning of social interaction and bonding.
- ➤ **Emotional Development:** Smiling is an essential part of a baby's emotional development. It reflects their ability to recognize and respond to positive experiences and emotions.

❖ **Capturing Memories: The Joy of Baby Photo Albums**

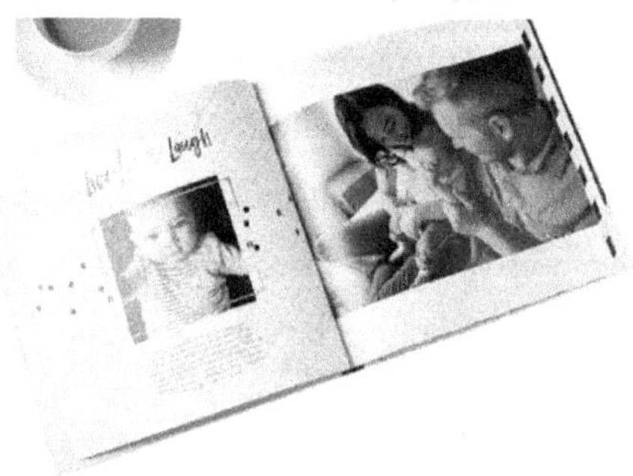

Time flies during parenthood, and before you know it, your baby will have grown into a toddler. Creating a baby photo album is a delightful way to cherish the precious moments and milestones you've shared together. Here are some tips for creating a memorable baby photo album:

- ➤ **Start early:** Begin documenting your baby's journey from the first day they come home. Capture everyday moments, such as bath time, playtime, and naptime, to show their growth and personality.
- ➤ **Include milestones:** Add images of important milestones like their first smile, first solid food, and first steps.
- ➤ **Personalize the album:** Add notes, captions, or anecdotes alongside the photos to preserve the emotions and memories associated with each image.
- ➤ **Digital vs. Print:** Decide whether you want a physical album or a digital one. Both options have their charms, so choose what suits your preferences best.

Parenthood is a remarkable journey filled with both challenges and rewarding moments. Embracing sleepless nights with patience and understanding will lead to beautiful moments like witnessing your baby's heartwarming smiles. Creating lasting memories through photo albums will allow you to cherish these precious times for years to come, making parenthood an unforgettable and cherished experience.

Conclusion

Delving into the intricate tapestry of pregnancy reveals a mesmerizing array of fascinating facts and insights surrounding expectant mothers. From the awe-inspiring biological processes that shape new life to the emotional and psychological transformations experienced by mothers-to-be, the journey of pregnancy is a profound and deeply human experience.

Throughout this exploration, we have uncovered the remarkable resilience and adaptability of the female body as it nurtures and sustains the development of a new being. We have also witnessed the immeasurable bond that forms between mother and child, even before birth, and the enduring impact it has on both their lives.

Furthermore, this journey into the world of expectant mothers has underscored the importance of comprehensive prenatal care, supportive environments, and a societal commitment to empower women during this transformative time. As we embrace scientific advancements and empathetic understanding, we can better navigate the complexities of pregnancy and provide the nurturing environment that every mother and child deserve.

As the web of knowledge surrounding pregnancy continues to expand, it is crucial that we remain ever-curious and compassionate, fostering an environment of continuous learning and support for expectant mothers. Only by acknowledging and celebrating the wonders and challenges of pregnancy can we truly appreciate the miraculous nature of human life and ensure the well-being of future generations.

In essence, the revelations surrounding pregnancy are not merely a collection of intriguing facts but a testament to the incredible beauty and strength inherent in the journey of motherhood. By cherishing and understanding this profound experience, we enrich the fabric of humanity and sow the seeds of a brighter and more compassionate future for all.

www.ingramcontent.com/pod-product-compliance
Lightning Source LLC
Chambersburg PA
CBHW071119260726
48661CB00006B/2648